YES YOU CAN

A GUIDE TO EXERCISE FOR BEGINNERS

MIKE WOMER

PRO PLAYER PUBLISHING
WILMINGTON, DE

Pro Player Publishing
300 Delaware Avenue, Suite 210
Wilmington, DE 19801
www.ProPlayerPress.com

Book Layout ©2013 BookDesignTemplates.com

Ordering Information:
Quantity sales. Special discounts are available on quantity purchases by corporations, associations, and others. For details, contact the "Special Sales Department" at the address above.

YES You Can! A Guide to Exercise for Beginners / Mike Womer. —1st ed.
ISBN 978-0-9814710-2-0

Dedication

I need to thank my wonderful wife who supports me regardless of
my endless lists of misadventures and constant state of chaos. What
kind of woman signs on to be married to a man who is convinced that
he is Peter Pan, is self employed, worked as a Pro Wrestler for over
twenty five years and seems to be constantly adding to his list of over
twenty surgeries. Did I mention "the boys"? Those are my friends
who clearly have a penchant for fun filled adventures.

So I dedicate this book to Sandy for her constant dedication to our
family, to me, my lifestyle and even my friends. I can't imagine this
journey without you – I love you to the moon!

Maybe the greatest thing about writing this book is that anything
I say about my son or to my son, Jake, will last forever.

Being Jake's dad is the greatest honor a man can ever have. Jake,
you are the most wonderful little boy I have ever seen.
I love you to bits!

CONTENTS

Preface

Over the years, clients have asked for me to share my health and fitness message via newsletters, texts, or emails. I'm an old school guy. I don't even have a Facebook account.

I've finally decided to embrace technology and start sharing my message through podcasts focused on helping beginners embrace a healthy lifestyle. This book summarizes those podcasts and shares simple steps YOU can take today to make the lifestyle changes YOU want.

If you have ever questioned whether you have what it takes to live the life you desire, this book answers- YES, YOU CAN!

Mike Womer
Newark, DE
January 2015

Acknowledgements

LEARNING THE "WELLNESS" BUSINESS

A ruptured patella tendon changed my journey from one seemingly well-defined path to the great unknown. That "unknown" led me to Paul Schweizer and Vaughn Bolton.

According to my surgeon my knee was the worst he had ever seen and would require extensive rehabilitation. The tendon that connects the bottom of my knee cap to the lower part of my knee broke loose and was pulled up into my thigh by my quad muscle. My surgeon told me that I was going to have a brutal rehab process and that I would need to accept a lot of discomfort. After surgery, I was sent to begin physical therapy at Paul Schweizer's facility.

After a day of rest, with stitches and staples still in my knee, I made my first visit to Schweizer's physical therapy. Immediately, I was told that I needed to wait at home until the wound healed completely and the staples were removed. I then began to plead my case – I just plain begged them to take me early. Begrudgingly they agreed.

My initial evaluation was with Paul, one of the most intense men on the planet and then I was sent to work with Vaughn, a man with the strength of a bull and the hands of a saint.

He and Paul worked on me and refused to accept anything less than my knee returning to 100%. I spent hours hooked to Vaughn's

v

torture device designed to force me to regain my range of motion and in the pool with Paul when the device didn't work well enough. Electric stim units hummed seemingly forever to speed up the process. The process was slow and was indeed filled with more pain then at that time I had ever experienced.

Unfortunately my many hours in rehab had extinguished all my allotted insurance visits. I asked Paul if he would give me movements and exercises to do on my own as my insurance had run out. Paul looked at me with a combination of disbelief and disgust. Without changing his expression he asked me if my knee was 100%. After I told him that my knee was not, he responded: "I'll see you Monday morning". He promptly got up and walked away. I immediately asked Vaughn what I should do, after all, I no longer had any visits left from insurance and I was not close to being better. Vaughn then begins to laugh at me and then strongly suggests that I arrive on time Monday.

And so it was–they treated me until I was better: for free. But that wasn't the greatest gift that those two gentlemen gave me. I learned more from Paul and Vaughn about human anatomy/bio-mechanics and how to get clients better then they will ever know. So much of what I do and how I act was learned from watching them in the original Schweizer's physical therapy.

1614 is full of ideas that I borrowed (stole) from Paul and Vaughn – thank you for your guidance and care.

WRITING A BOOK!

I want to thank Chuck Boyce and all the people at Pro Player Publishing who thought that our message and many silly stories deserved to be published. I could not have done it without you. I hope I haven't driven you too crazy. I promise one of these days I will give in and just comb my hair!!

Insanity: doing the same thing over and over and expecting different results.

Albert Einstein

[1]

Yes You Can

I HEAR THIS ALL the time, "Do you know that Debbie ran a 5K," or "Chuck ran a triathlon," or "Dino did the mud run, but me? I could never do that."

I hear that all the time: "I could never do that."

My question is, why? Why can't you do it?

Let's talk about what I think you really want to say.

When somebody says to me, "I can't do that," I really believe in my heart that what you should say is either "I've never done that before", or "I don't really want to do that," because I think if you want to do it, I bet you can.

I get up every day at 4:30 a.m. I'm an early bird, not by choice, but just because life happens that way.

Have you ever done what I call the clock prayer? This morning I'm laying in bed, and I've got the drool coming out. I'm so excited; I'm happy. I wake up for some stupid reason and then I immediately go into the clock prayer. The clock prayer is when you say, "Please, God, Please, God, make it be midnight, make it be midnight."

I looked at the clock this morning. My alarm is set to go off at 4:30. It's 4:22. That's bad. That's terrible. That is not a way to start the day.

So I lay there a few more minutes. The drool is now dried. I'm cranky, and I figure, "What the heck. Let me just get up."

Nine times out of 10 I beat the alarm, because I'm cursed, but it is what it is. When people hear me say I get up at 4:30, they're like, "Dude, what? Why would you ever get up at 4:30?"

One time I was going fishing with this dude. He was a little bit older than me. He says, "Listen. We'll meet somewhere for coffee at 6:30. Is that too early for you?"

I'm like, "Dude, no. I'll be there." He questions, and questions, and questions. I'm like, "I'll be there."

Long story short, I get up at 4:30 every day, and people all the time say, "Dude, I could never do that."

"I could never do that." Let's go back to what I said a few seconds ago, "I've never done that before," or "I don't want to do that." I think it's one of the two, because I think you can get up.

READY TO CHANGE

Unfortunately, life creates situations where we have to react when we don't really want to. It might be getting sick, getting injured, or sometimes worse, a loved one gets sick or injured. We see people go through awful life experiences that they don't want to go through, but they have to. They then make dramatic life changes, not because they want to, they have to make the changes. These are remarkable people; and they make amazing changes.

"I could never do that."

Unfortunately, those people have no choice.

Remember those people who say they can't do it, "I could never run a 5K. I could never do a triathlon. I could never do a mud run. I could never get up at 4:30."

Either you've never done it before, or you just don't want to. If you want to do something, you can.

One of my favorite phrases, and it's grammatically disastrous, but I love it,

"You always do what you've always done, you always get what you've always got."

Right now, Mr. Romano my grammar teacher in high school is rolling over, because that grammatically is a disaster.

"You always do what you've always done, you always get what you've always got." I know, it's terrible, but it's true, isn't it?

If you want to do something different, you've got to change. You can't have change without distilling some sort of change.

Insanity: doing the same thing over and over again and expecting different results. – Albert Einstein

What's the greatest example of insanity? Doing the same act over and over and over and over and expecting a different result. It's just not going to happen. "I could never do that." If you were to do that, you've got to change things. You've got to change things pretty dramatically. "I can't get up at 4:30." That's a mouthful, "I can't get up at 4:30." They're emphatic, too, by the way. They want to know I can't possibly get up then. That's crazy.

PAULA

Let me tell you a story. I'm going to give you 3 examples of people who can, they were dealt a card, or hand of cards, much worse and much

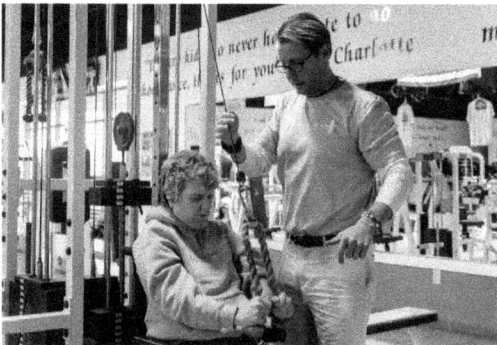

more challenging than I'm ever going to get.

Let's start with Paula. Paula doesn't have use of anything from below her mid-torso. Paula has been training at 1614 for 12 years... 12

years!

I get up, get a shower, put on my socks and shoes, put on my shirt, drive to the gym, act like a buffoon, have my coffee, act like a buffoon, say "Hello," act like a buffoon... I know; it's a trend. Bottom line is, I get to do all these things easily and comfortably. I walk into the gym and I work out.

Nothing Paula does is easy. I've never in 12 years, heard her complain about it and I see her all the time. She couldn't come to the gym this week, because she's got a sore on her leg. She's got complications, because of he wheelchair chair. But I will guarantee she'll be there next week.

Think about that. People say they can't go to the gym. Paula's not in the gym this week because she's got a sore on her leg, but she'll be there next week.

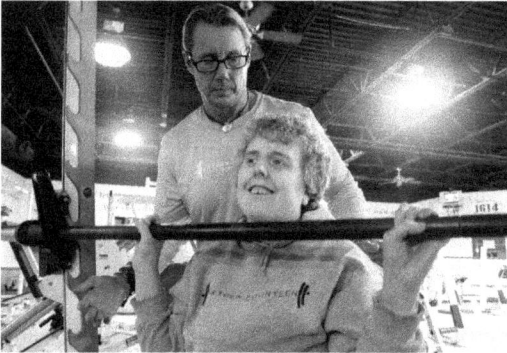

"I can't get up at 4:30." That's crazy.

All right. Let's go back to Paula. Paula's in a wheelchair, so for Paula to work out we have to make some adjustments. For example the Smith machine is this apparatus with rods and it's basically a bench press or cage, but it's in a supported rack. Anyway, normally we would use a bench, but Paula can't get on the bench. So we lock her down and we actually use her wheelchair as a bench, and she works out.

She can bench press. She does close grip. Then we get her up, we spin her around, she checks her pretty self out in the mirror, and she does shoulder presses.

She's in a wheelchair, people, with a hurt leg.

When we're done that, we cruise over and we do dumbbell raises. I tell her she's flapping like a bird, and I just say something mean and nasty. She loves it and gives it right back to me. I pick on her constantly.

Then we cruise around to a pulley station and we do triceps pushdowns, all of which is being facilitated while she is in a wheelchair.

I have people look at me all the time, "I can't get up at 4:30."

Really?

Paula got herself up, dressed, cleaned, got on DART, got off DART, came in the gym, and worked out.

God bless her. Paula can do it. She does it all the time.

Paula. Thank you.

AUSTIN

Which brings me to Austin. If the story of this young man doesn't give you chills, you're done, man.

Here he is.

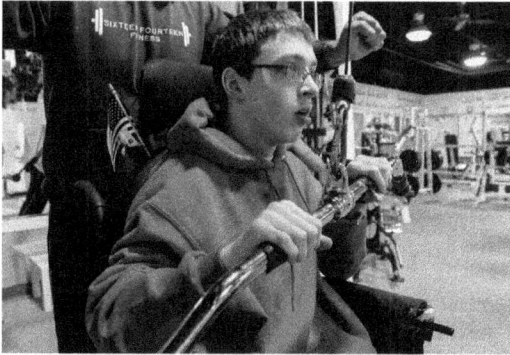

We call him Dude Love, because he's just a dude and he's a lot of fun. He's a high school student going to school locally. He's also in a chair. Bottom line, his body doesn't react the way ours does. Everything's kind of tightened up.

If you don't understand men, and a lot of people don't, I can tell you one fact. At one point in a man's/boy's life, we all want to bench press. Some it lasts for years and years; others it lasts for 10 minutes. At one point or another every boy wants to bench press.

I got to know this young man, through my nephew. We were talking, and this and that, and he's got this ear to ear grin, and he says to me, "You know, I've always wanted to bench press, but I just can't do it."

Me, being the buffoon that I am, says, "Why not?"

He looks at me, "What do you mean, why not?"

I said, "Well, why can't you?"

He goes, "Dude ..."

"I thought that we could figure it out."

He says, "Really?"

"I don't know what we'd do, or even how we'd do it, but maybe ..."

He says, "Can I try?"

Now I've painted myself in a corner. I'd better figure it out. I said, "Meet me at the gym at 6:00 on Thursday," and his mom is foolish enough to bring him.

They bring him, and I don't know what to do. His chair is different than Paula's. It's got parts on it that I don't understand. I asked his mom, "What am I allowed to do to this child?"

Her reply, "I don't care. I'm doing cardio."

"For real?" I said, "Did you sign this form?"

She says, "Yes."

I said, "Sign it again."

"Okay."

She signed it 5 times, because I know I'm going to get sued. I said, "Are you sure I can do anything?"

She says, "I'm doing cardio. Leave me alone."

He's looking at me like this, "Are we benching?"

"Son, I don't know what we're going to do, but we're going to try."

I scoop him up and I lay him on the bench. He begins to wiggle.

"You're going to fall off." I take my belt off and strap his duff to the bench.

People are looking at me, "What is he doing?"

"I'm strapping him to the bench with my belt." Then I pull away and go, "I'm going to kick you now, watch," and he starts giggling and laughing.

I have Austin strapped to the bench, and his hands don't want to go where they want to go, but we figure it out.

He benches. He looked up at me and he started to shake. He was so excited that he benched. He was out of his mind.

"Dude, was that cool, or what?"

He was so excited, genuinely excited out of his mind. Take yourself back to high school. For me it's 122 years ago, but take yourself back. There's a huge period of that where all that matters is that you're cool, cool in one group. There's all these groups now. You want to be cool with one of them.

If you roll into school in a wheelchair, it's going to be tough to be cool. It don't matter to me. I don't think it ever mattered to me that much, but to kids it does. Here's a dude who's in a chair in high school, who comes to a gym. He told me, "I was scared to death." Now he's so excited that he's in a gym and he's benched like a big boy. He's shaking.

Before long, he starts coming in every week. Before long, all of the guys in the gym knew him and they all talked to him.

He's puffing up, "Hey, what's up? I'm benching today." He started doing the gym nod, too ... made me happy.

He will be there. He's there twice a week with his mom. His mom now, she gets up and helps me. I have a belt in my office that I use to strap him down.

I'm proud.

I'm happy.

We did this. I'm thinking we're done. We're benching and we're doing different things. Again, physically we've got some challenges. We've got to work around something, but he does every time.

Then there's people who say, "I can't get up at 4:30." Okay.

Then he looks at me ... Austin looks at me and says, "You know what I've always wanted to do?" Now he's cocky, because he's in a gym. He gets all puffy. "You know what I've always wanted to do? I've always wanted to use the leg press."

"What? Just shut up and bench."

"No. I think I can leg press."

"Mom, he wants to leg press."

She said, "Well, go ahead."

"You've got to sign more forms. There's a lot of forms you need to sign, and I need notary, or whatever that is. I need pictures ... Shut up! ... Sign. Stamp it."

So I said, "For real, can he ...? I don't know what capacity these legs are, so we just have to be careful. I'm legitimately terrified that I'm going to hurt him."

He asks, "How are we going to do it?" and I don't have a clue.

I pick him up, we get him back in his chair, and we go over to the leg press. We have a quasi-horizontal leg press.

I pick him up. We got him in the leg press. He's seated. He's sitting kind of upright. I said, "Buddy, hold on. Hold on. There's handles here." I said, "I'm serious now. I'm a goofball, but safety is paramount in my world. Please hold on, buddy."

He knows I'm serious, because I get that look, "Hold on." He's holding on, and then eventually I said, "Mom, get over here and hold him," and I start going to get props.

I go get that belt. I strap him, and then I hold his legs up. I've got his feet here, and now I've got my leg here, and I'm literally spotting him with my foot.

I look like I'm playing Twister on a piece of equipment. It's ridiculous. He's giggling and laughing. "Don't laugh, son. You'll fall the hell off. Just stay still." Even before he tries to press, his knees kick in.

"Hold on. I'll be right back." I run to my office. Now I come back with a ball. I got a little play ball, so I put it between his legs, and we're going to keep his knees from caving in.

I've got his feet. I've got my leg holding up. I said, "Let's go. Let's go." He moves it just a smidge ... that much, puts it down, and his eyes go, Whoo! He goes, "I did it."

I said, "Bro, I know you did," and he did it again, and he did it again, and he did it again. He did it and he went into that shake. Oh! He liked leg presses.

This is a dude who wheels into school, wheels into the gym, benches, and then drops the leg press thing on me. That's amazing. If Austin doesn't inspire you, you're dead. He's a rock star.

So if you can't get up at 4:30, I still believe you've never done it before.

"I don't really want to do that." I think that's a more truthful statement. I'm not a big karma guy, but I do believe you've got to be true to others as well as yourself.

If you say you can't do it, and you really can, isn't that lying to yourself? I just think that creates a bad mojo that I don't want any part of. I'd much rather say I'd never done it before, or "I don't want any part of it."

Truth be told, I don't want to get up at 4:30, but I do.

JOHNNY

Hold on. I've got one more. I've got Paula; I've got Austin. I've got one more ... Johnny.

Johnny's got a condition that's got a whole lot of letters. It's big. He's a sweetheart I've known him for about 20 years.

John's in a chair, but not all the time. This condition that he has is ultimately, to really simplify it ... His joints are twisted, scrunched a little bit, and they just don't cooperate. His body doesn't cooperate, but his soul and his mind very much wants to cooperate. He wants to do everything, and God bless him for it.

John says, similar to Dude Love, he says, "Mike, I want to do cardio." I'm thinking, "Cardio ..." Again, I don't know the capacity of his knees and legs, so I said, "What can you do? What do you think?"

He says, "Let's try getting on the EFX." I'm nervous Nellie again. The character Mike Womer's a silly rabbit, but I'm a serious guy when it comes to safety.

I said, "You want to get up there and do this?" I don't know if he can do it. We get him up there. Again, his joints don't work in a fluid motion like ours do. None of them work in a fluid motion. He's on the EFX, and parts are moving, and I'm moving.

He's excited. I'm worried, and he's happy.

"Are you all right?"

He's smiles, "Oh, yeah. I'm good. Oh, I'm good." We get him down and we go through our workout, and he becomes committed, committed to the gym.

Think about it. If you're in a chair, your physical needs are different in terms of what you have to do, you have to transfer in and out of the wheelchair. There are just different demands on your body to compensate for the day-to-day things that you need to do.

From a physical perspective, there's some exercises that you can do to help make your life easier. John really wanted to work on his shoulders and his chest. He loved the chest. He'd do bench and he'd pound on his chest and grin at me. So he did that.

He also said, "I really want to lose some weight, so let's get back on the EFX." We're on the EFX and we're moving and we're moving. He's working like a champ.

One day I get a text. He stated that his hips are really hurting. I just heard, "hurt" ... "Oh, no. John hurt himself. We finally pushed John a little too far. Not good."

I pick him up and I call. I know I called, because I was worried. I said, "John, what's going on?"

He goes, "Oh, my gosh. It hurts so bad."

I'm like, "Aw, man. This is bad. All right, where?"

"It's not my back so much. It's not my back of the legs. It's my bum, the meat of my bum. It's ... it's on fire."

"The meat part of your bum?"

"Yes!"

"John, that's your butt muscle."

"So, that's a good thing, right?"

"Yes! It's actually a great thing."

John hasn't turned on his glutes, maybe for the first time ever. He described it as, "Mike, my butt's on fire!"

"Dude, that's great news. That's like me or somebody else doing squats. We turned your glutes on for the first time, and they're reacting. You've got blood flow; you've got hamstrings working; you've got stuff going on back there. God bless you, brother."

Let's go back to the original point I'm making. "Mike, you get up at 4:30? Chuck, you're doing a mud run? Dino, you're doing a 5K?"

"I can't do that. That's impossible. I can't do that. I can't do that."

Paula gets up every day, gets herself in a chair. Dude Love benches, goes to school every day. Johnny gets on an EFX out of his chair, and now walks across the gym in front of everybody, showing off. Isn't that fun?

People tell me, "I can't get up at 4:30."

Lucky for you, I can help that.

I can solve that problem forever.

Here it is. First of all, the snooze button is a complete waste of time. It's all a lie. Remember that pretty girl who said she was going to go roller skating with you back in the seventh grade, but never did? That was a lie. Snooze button is a dirty, awful lie.

Here's what happens with the snooze button: you hit it; it stays quiet for 7 minutes. When you shut your eyes, 13 seconds later it's going off, "Waa, waa, waa," and you hit it again. Now you're frustrated and you're late.

Not good.

Here's what you do. You're laying in bed; the alarm clock goes off. Guess what? You stand up. I know, crazy thinking, right? Stand up. Then you turn off your alarm, and here's what's going to happen: either a) you're going to wake up or b) you're going to fall asleep and fall down.

When you fall down, you're going to wake up anyway. Then you get a shower and everything's good.

Anybody can get up at 4:30.

Anybody can make change.

The problem is, we've got to believe it. "You always do what you've always done, you always get what you've always got." It's simple.

Paula chose not to do what she's always done. Austin chose not to do what he's always done. Johnny, same story.

If you say you can't, maybe it's your approach. Maybe you've just got to accept that you've never done it before, or you don't really want to.

If you haven't done it before, and you do want to, now we're cooking. Now you've got an opportunity to change your life. If you have something that you want, but you've never done it before, it certainly doesn't mean that you can't do it. It just means that you need to instill change in your current life to allow you to do it, just like those folks did: Paula, Austin, and John.

All those folks decided they wanted something that they never did before that, quite frankly, was a much bigger leap than getting up at 4:30, which is a much bigger leap than running a mud run, a much bigger leap than doing a 5K.

5Ks, and mud runs, and 4:30...That's cake.

Those people I talked about before, they're doing something special. If you have something that you truly want to do, but just haven't done it before, what you need then is a plan to establish a game plan so you can go do it.

Next we are going to talk about Goals. If you want that thing, but have never done it before, you've got to come up with a game plan to make it happen.

"You always do what you've always done, you'll always get what you've always got."

These folks I keep talking about here, Paula, Austin, and John, they changed and they got what they wanted, and you can, too. It's all a matter of understanding what it is that you want and coming up with a plan.

[2]

Goals

WHY DO I FEEL SO STRONGLY about goals? I think goals can help make people happier. I think goals can improve one's position in life and work. I just think it keeps you moving. For me, movement is hugely important. I'm a big fan of that. I'll share with you why.

Our body, depending on who you talk to, is comprised of 60-80% water. I think there are some parallels there between our body and water.

Moving water creates life, creates life at the cellular level. It absolutely provides an environment where things can live and breathe and the food chain can begin or end. Also, that moving water helps create energy. Back at the very beginning of our country, settlements huddled around rivers and streams. It creates life. Moving water is precious.

Water that stays still, stagnant, can kill you. It can foster an environment that is the antitheses of life. It is absolutely dreadful. Moving water: great. Stagnant water: dreadful.

The human body, the same thing really. If you sit down, just sit down in a chair and don't move, within 48 hours, your body begins to atrophy.

Atrophy is just a fancy word of breaking down. You will begin to break down muscle tissue. You will begin to become weaker and softer. Really, you're truly breaking down at the molecular level. You're falling apart. Conversely, if you run, if you move, if you remain active, your body and your life and your health can flourish.

Moving water: good. Moving body: good. Stagnant body, stagnant water: dreadful.

I'm a firm believer that if you set goals, you're going to move. You're going to go places you might not otherwise go.

Let's create some goals.

One of my favorite lines is "If you're not going somewhere, you're going nowhere". It sounds a little elementary, I guess, but it's true. If I don't have someplace to go, what am I doing? I'm not going anywhere. A better quote, maybe, is from Andrew Carnegie.

If you want to be truly happy, select a goal that commands your thoughts, liberates your energies, and inspires your hopes. – Andrew Carnegie

That's a mouthful that I wish I came up with. Doesn't that really embody everything I'm trying to say to you? It's just absolutely a fantastic thought. If you have a goal, it's going to create a ton of opportunities for your thought, your spirits, your mind.

Here is something that happens to me all the time.

I'm a trainer. Folks come in. They want me to train them. They come in all geared up. They got their water bottle. They got their sneakers. They got their sweats. They got their shirts. They're all ready to go.

The first thing I say to them is, "Hey come on, let's go meet and talk in my office." You can see the "Eh" in their eyes because they were excited to work out and they can't for the life of them figure out why I don't want to work out.

I don't.

I want to sit and talk.

They quickly think that this is a monster waste of time. Right from the giddy up, I think this is the most significant thing that we're going to do in terms of our relationship. We sit down and we talk. The first thing I want to know is what is it that you want to do?

They start talking and they start talking. I'm convinced from years and years of marketing and TV ads and cereals that are going to help you do this and bars that are going to help you do this and new weight this and that, they immediately say, "I'm going to lose 20 pounds."

I don't know whether they really want that or they just want to shut me up so we can get out there and work out. Regardless, that's what they say. Through it all, I keep talking and I keep talking and I keep talking because I want to know what really it is that they want.

Here is a specific story about a woman I met a long time ago. We were doing just that. We were sitting down, we're talking and we're going over her goals and this and that. She also, wanted to lose 20 pounds.

I knew that wasn't that significant. I kept talking to her and talking to her. Before long, I realized there was a trend. She kept bringing up a trip. She kept bringing up her husband. She kept bringing up a bikini. I said, "Listen, I hear the 20 pounds, but what is it that you really want?"

Then, I challenged her. I hear your husband, I hear bikini, I hear trip. What is it that you want? She immediately became emotional and began to cry. She says, "Mike, we've been married for," I don't remember this, 15 years maybe, "I've never once wore a bikini in front of my husband. We're going away in three months and I'd love nothing more than a chance to wear that bikini."

"Hun, there is your goal. That right there is a perfect goal. That goal will motivate you and inspire you to get out of bed and work.

That goal will motivate and inspire you to do things that you might not be willing to do for that scale."

Losing 20 pounds, that's great and losing 20 pounds may get her in that bikini, but sometimes, you need something more tangible to get your arms around to motivate you to make it happen.

We wrote it down. We did all that good stuff and when it was all said and done, she made her goal. She sent me a picture of her in that red bikini, with her husband on a beach somewhere. I really don't believe that if the goal would have been 20 pounds, it would have happened.

Enough about her. What is a goal? A lot of folks think they have goals. I just think they're desires or whims. That's what I call them. They might be shown as, "You know what, I think I'm going to run a 5K." "You know what, I'm going to lose that 20 pounds," or "I think I might go back and get my degree." I think those are desires or whims. They're just thoughts that pop into my head, that really haven't turned into more than that.

The question is how do you turn a whim or a desire into a goal?

WRITE IT DOWN

First thing you got to do is you have to give it life. You have to make it tangible. You got to make it real. For me, we're going to do just what she did. We're going to write it down. Write that goal down and make it real, make it tangible. Make it something you can hold. Don't just write it down once, write it down a couple different times and put it in places. Put it places that you're going to see it everyday.

I call them life intersections. A life intersection might be a refrigerator. Might be the dash of your car. Might be your computer terminal. Put it in places that you'll see it. We all know that old phrase, "Out of sight, out of mind," and let's face it, that's true. If you don't think about it, you don't see it, it just goes away. Magically, it's gone.

Conversely, if I put it in sight, it's going to tend to stay in mind. Put that goal in strategic places. Your mirror in your bathroom. Your dash of your car. All these places you're going to see it. Keep it in front of you. Make it real. We're going to give it life. We're going to turn it on by writing it down. That's a great step, but that's still not a goal in my world. That's still not what we need to do because we'll go back to my friend.

She had a goal of getting into a bikini on the vacation date. What we have to do is now take that goal and create urgency. Give it urgency by giving a date. That's huge.

If I have an open ended goal, "I'm going to run a 5K," don't have a date in mind, I just want to run a 5K, the likelihood of that happening isn't so great because there is no urgency to it.

URGENCY

Urgency is key. Ask any parent or teacher that's tried to get a child to do a book report. Sense of urgency is huge in getting it done. Typically, they're going to start that homework the day before. That's not going to work.

Write down the goal, "I'm going to run a 5K October 22nd" and then sign your name to it. Now, it has life. I've written it down. I've established urgency. I've put a date and I sign it. Now, I've got that set out all around my home. All over the place so I see it and it becomes absolutely truly real. Now, we've got a challenge. Now, it seems as though everything we needed is done.

My goal is set. I want to run a 5K by October 22nd. That's my goal. Not quite. We have to validate it. We've got to see how badly I want this goal.

My gal that I worked with earlier, she wanted it badly. It brought up emotion. There were tears involved. That's a wonderful goal because I know there is an emotional buy-in. It goes back to the scale, there is no emotional buy-in with that scale. It's ridiculous. Unless you're Flavor Flav and going wear it around your neck, it's insignificant. I need emotional buy-in.

When I have my clients do their goal, I go, "Great, on a scale of one to 10, how badly do you want this goal? One being eh, 10 being I want it so badly I can taste it."

Hers was a ten. I knew we were going to get it. I knew she would do what she had to do. So much so, I asked her to buy that bikini and secretly hang it in her closet just to keep that motor going.

How badly do you want it? You have to validate your goal so you know if you're lying to yourself or not.

COMMITMENT TO CHANGE

Think about it. I may think I want it, but for me to run a 5K or me to go do something drastic requires change. You can't expect to have change without implementing change in your life. We, as people, don't always like change. Change is kind of scary, it's uncomfortable. Think about it, some of the best or most popular TV shows were the ones that did the same thing over and over and over and over. Change, for a lot of people, isn't welcome.

You have to ask yourself, "Do I really want it?" Here is a quick story about a young man who wanted desperately, he thought, to go back and get his degree. At the time, he had a good job, had spending money, had free time where he could work a couple hours at a bar, had extra money so he could drive around in his sports car, and he thought to himself, "This is fantastic."

He didn't get his degree and he realized some of the folks he originally went to school with had gotten their degree and were passing him professionally. That caused him to say to himself, maybe on a whim, "I got to go back and get my degree." He goes. He even writes it down. He even comes up with a date, but he never validated it. He never asked himself how badly does he want it.

He goes back, takes a couple classes, finishes those, does well, takes a couple more.

All of a sudden, that extra financial cushion that he had is gone because he can't work as much. He can't work the extra job. He's got to pay for books. He's got to pay for the classes themselves. All of a sudden, he's running out of money. But he can't work those extra hours anymore because he's got to study. This is becoming ugly.

He can't really afford that sports car anymore because all of the reasons I just mentioned. Now, all of a sudden, he no longer works at that cool bar, he no longer has a sports car, and he's doing studies and homework all the time.

Few months into this process, he decided maybe that's not what he wanted and he jumped off the ship before it got too deep. He went back and got his other job, got himself another car. He realized he didn't want it that badly.

The gal who got a bikini on, she did. I'm a firm believer to truly make a goal, you have to give it life. Write it down. Write it down and put it all over the place. Life's intersections. Put it in places that you're going to see it. Give it a date. Give it urgency. First, you have to give it life, then you got to give it urgency, then you have to have your come to Jesus, I call it. How badly do I want it? Because you're never going to have change without change.

I love that definition of insanity. Insanity is when you do the same thing over and over and over and over and keep expecting a different result. It doesn't happen. You have to ask yourself, "Am I truly willing to accept those changes to reach my goal?" We have goals in my office, I often ask folks, "Listen, how badly do you want this goal, one or 10?" They hem and they haw. I say, "Listen, cut to the chase. Is this goal significant enough for you to get out of your bed on a cold, rainy

November Saturday at 7:30 in the morning to come into the gym and do cardio? Is it?" They go, "Yeah." And I say, "No, no, is it really?"

I can see them thinking. If the answer is yes, we have got ourselves a very good goal. If not, it's probably not going to work. How do you make a goal come to life? You have to give it life by writing it down. Then, you have to give it urgency by giving it a due date. Then, you have to validate it and find out how badly you want it. Are you willing to make the sacrifices necessary to make this goal come true? If you are, then we're set.

The only other piece of advice I want to give you on the urgency aspect is if you've got a goal that's this big, that's more than three, four, five, six months in duration, I encourage you to cut it up into small chunks. Establish workable parts. If you do those three things, give it life, give it a sense of urgency, and then validate it, I think you're well on your way to movement and keeping yourself happy.

That's how we do those goals. I like to offer a quick tidbit in conclusion. I want to give you three characteristics of what I think make up a great goal. I think every goal needs to move you. I think it should move you emotionally. I think it should move you physically. I think it should move you cognitively.

Let's talk about that real quickly. I do think a goal should move you physically. You should get up and move around. I don't think you necessarily have to have every goal has to be a 5K, an exercise this, an exercise that, but I hope it requires you to get up and move. I hope it requires to get up and make blood flow. I hope it makes you go from point A to point B because I guarantee you in a weird way, that will make you feel better. I hope it moves you physically.

I also hope it moves you emotionally. I hope it is something so significant, at the end of it, you can sit down and feel good about it. Whether or not it's tears over a bikini, whether or not it's finishing a 5K, whether or not it's going back to get your degree, whether it's getting that promotion, I hope it is serious enough that it causes emotion.

Finally, I think it should move you cognitively. Every goal we have needs to make us think. We have got to think. We have got to establish plans. It has got to be significant enough where we have got to take a step back and create a plan. That plan needs to be organized and structured. It needs to fit into that whole game plan.

I do think a goal should move us physically, it should move us emotionally, it should move us cognitively.

[3]

4 + 1 = 5

"WHAT IN THE WORLD am I supposed to eat?"

So I've been doing this fitness thing for 15-16 years and truly the most common question that people give to me is this, "Mike, just tell me what to eat." Or this is a good one too. They'll look up on our rack of supplements and proteins and things of that nature and they'll go, "Look Mike, I know its right there, I know the secrets up there. Come on, give it to me." And these are guys that have been working out and gals who have been working out for years. And they are literally pointing up on our rack of supplements and they say, "Give me the secret."

There is no secret. There's absolutely no secret.

Let me show you a secret.

Those items that I just referred to? Supplements? That's short for supplemental. Those things are intended to supplement your diet. We'll talk about that in a little bit. But there is no secret. Reality is, it's all about life changing decisions. And that's exactly what this equation, 4+1=5 is all about. Yeah, I'm going to simplify nutrition and eating into that simple equation and let's start right now.

So let's think about it. Ultimately, what is the secret? We put food in, we exercise by taking food out, and we end up with our body. My body really is made up of two very important things: what I eat and what I do with my body. Those two things come together to give me my body. If I want to change my body, I need to change what I put into it and/or how I exercise. I feel silly saying that, but ultimately, that's the truth.

That being said, I explain that to people and they go, "OK great, that makes sense. So tell me what to eat." It doesn't work that way. It doesn't work that way at all and here's why. These fad diets have been around for 100 years and they're great at making money and I'm not so great at making money, but I'm pretty at helping people change their body. Those diets tell you what to eat. You can't be told every day what to eat. If I tell you to eat cabbage all day, every day and drink water, I guarantee you're going to lose weight like a champ. I also guarantee that you're not going to be happy with me and you're not going to do it for more than a couple days. So me telling you what to eat simply won't work.

Doug

We've got to figure some things out, so let me start this equation out by telling you a story. This story is about my buddy Doug. A long time ago I worked in corporate America and I'm sitting at my desk and this bang on the door. I look up and Doug comes in. I say, "Hey Doug, what's going on?" Honest to heaven this is what he said.

He said, "Boss, in case you haven't noticed, I'm fat. Been fat since I was a kid. In fact I went to fat camp. Fat camp didn't work so guess what? Still was a fat kid and I'm a fat adult."

I said, "Doug, you're not fat."

"I'm husky then."

"Regardless of what you are, what can I help you with?"

He says, "Listen. I know you do all this fitness stuff." Even before I started the gym I was known as a fitness guy. He says, "Can you help me?"

I said, "Sure buddy, I sure can."

At the time, in corporate America, I was teaching a finance class where I helped people save their money. Spend more efficiently. Be more aware of where their money was going. In that class, I had people write down everything that they spent their money on. Which is exactly what I did with people who are trying to eat better.

So that being said I reached under my desk and I grabbed him one of these little diary things. I threw it to him and I said, "Doug, write everything down that you eat. Everything that goes into your mouth write it down. Everything. Now get out of my office."

He grumbled and gruffed and stomped out. 3, 4, 5 days later, I can't remember, bang-bang-bang, I look up and there's Doug. He walks in, he throws this diary on my desk and it looks like it had been to Beirut and back. Bombed, ripped, torn, blown up, shot, everything.

"Well. Sit down. It looks as though you truly have taken this diary everywhere." I start reading it and I'm reading it and it didn't say one Cheetos or a bag of Cheetos, it said 14 Cheetos and it said, "I drank 1 beer, 2 beer." Then it got sloppier so I knew he was telling me the truth.

He did a great job.

"All right, great, now what's the secret?"

"Great here's the next thing." I reach under the desk, way 100 years ago we used books, not Google, Gaggle and all those other things. "Here bud. I need you to take this book, take everything that you're eating right now and quantify them."

"What's that mean boss?"

"Buddy I need you to figure out how many calories you're taking in. Every day. Then I need you to figure out how many grams of protein you're taking away. Every day. Fat and carbohydrates and that's it. Need you to go back and quantify all these days and as we move forward I need you to quantify those moving forward."

And he says, "Well do you want me to change?" Absolutely nothing, I don't want him to change. And the reason for not changing is simple. I want to know what's wrong.

When a mechanic fixes your car they need to get into the engine, under the hood. Regardless the type of car, they open the hood and look at it, figure out what's broken. Alternator, starter, whatever. Then, they can fix it. I need to get under his hood to figure out what's wrong.

"Listen. Take a week, quantify everything, get me numbers and come back and see me." So he did.

I realized very clearly that Doug was eating poorly. Not only was his caloric intake way high, but it was soft. Meaning they weren't calorically dense. Dense calories were coming from maybe vegetables, egg whites, lean meats, things of that nature. Low calories, high nutrition value, as opposed to high caloric intake, low nutrition value. We'll call those soft foods.

He had a ton of soft foods. Very, very little dense foods and from an exercise perspective, he wasn't doing anything. He wasn't going to a gym, he wasn't walking, and he wasn't actively playing a sport. He was working and going home and doing not much of anything.

So let's change our view here a little bit.

Let's take Doug and put him in this equation.

His food, or his 4, combined with what he was doing, very little, gave him that body. OK? Very simplified I know, this is very simple. That was his lifestyle and it gave him that body.

He says, "OK great so now what do we do?" I said, "If you want to change this, I'm going to use the C word again. If you want to change that 5, you've got to change preferably both of those, but at least one of those. We've got to make change."

I said, "Let's do this. Let's knock off 300 calories a day." I shared with him how we're going to do that. I made change. 300 calories. I said, "Listen, soon I'd like to see you make change in your exercise world."

He said, "Well what if I go where you go?"

"That'd be great."

At the time, next to 1614 Fitness the greatest gym I've ever seen in my life, High Energy in Newark.

"Come with me, we'll get you doing cardio. 15 minutes a day, 3 days a week."

So we reduced his calories, we increased his activity level, which in turn will change his body.

He replied, very excited, "Oh my goodness when is this going to change, when will this change occur?"

Well here's something that's pretty neat.

I've read study after study. Typically when people make a life change, such as Doug, it takes 30-40 days to see the difference. When people join a gym, typically they stay 20-30 days before they bail. So in other words, when those guys do those New Year's Resolutions, they join in January, they go about 19, 18 or 17, 18, 19, 20 days and they go, "Pfft, this isn't working." They bail. Well unfortunately they bailed about 10 days before their body is going to make change. I said,

"Doug, give it 2 months." I thought for sure it'd happen before that but I go, "Give it 2 months." So he did. We came back and revisited that, his book was very thorough. He did indeed reduce his calories by 300. He manipulated that number and he indeed lost.

Now, why did I have him write it down? Well it's 2 reasons really. We need to figure out what's wrong by getting under the hood so that was important. I can help somebody achieve long term success as opposed to a fad diet quick fix that won't last. I can help somebody have a long-term success if we modify their current eating habits as opposed to completely reshaping everything.

If I have a guy and a vegetarian and I'm going to ask him to eat lean chicken that's a train wreck, that's ridiculous. I would much rather see the eating habits of a client, modify it gradually as opposed to just scrambling everything up and changing everything. That I think is a recipe for disaster whereas here, I think we've got a very good chance of success.

All right, so let's get back to things.

We lowered his calories by 300, we increased his calories. We increased his activity level. His body changed.

"All right Doug, it's time to make another move."

"OK I'm assuming we're going to lose some more calories, right?"

"We're going to change your calories."

Remember I mentioned soft calories versus dense calories?

"All right bud, now the real work begins. You need to eat like an athlete."

He looks at me and goes, "Boss, do I look like an athlete to you?"

"Yeah, you are an athlete. You've moving your body, aren't you? You're trying to make your body perform aren't you? That's what an athlete does in my world. It doesn't mean you're on TV, doesn't mean you're in the Olympics, but you're an athlete and you need to eat that way."

We went over the exercise, "Take a look at this sliced lunch meat. Look at the calories there. What if we get rid of that and what if you decide to make some lean chicken breast Sunday and bring them in with brown rice? Same calories, but a lot denser by doing it yourself and probably more financially sound as well."

He did that. It took work. It took effort. Which a lot of people aren't necessarily willing to do, but he was. So he did. And you know what? We revisited him again. He lost more weight.

"What's next, boss?" So then we gradually bumped up his cardio. We went from 15 three days a week to 20 three days a week to 20 four days a week to eventually he started lifting weights.

Long story short, we made additional adjustments so by time this story was finished, he was eating cleanly. I'm going to say all the time but I'm going to give you a wink and I'll get back to that in a second, but he was eating cleanly all the time, working out very aggressively, and his body? He dropped 65 pounds.

This is the guy who assured me "fat farm" wouldn't work, doctors his mother sent him to didn't work, and everything he tried didn't work.

I understood.

I truly believe in my heart of heart that the body is a mathematical equation. Now if we've got an illness and we're taking drugs, we've got side effects, that's a whole different animal. But if things are working, I hate to say the word correctly or normally, this equation is going to work a lot more times than it fails. Truth be told, I've never done it with a client that it didn't work. Because isn't that the basis? That's our food coming in, that's our food coming out, and that's what's left. If we manipulate these two variables the end result is going to be different.

All right so let's go back to the wink, wink when I said Doug ate well all the time. If you think for a second that I don't enjoy happy hour and wings and pizza, you're out of your mind. You're out of your mind.

People look at me and they go, "Oh you're the fitness guy. You eat cardboard and broccoli all the time." I do eat my share of broccoli. I've never eaten cardboard and everybody feels guilty. They always walk to me and they go,

"Dude, I had a piece of pizza the other day."

"Dude, I don't care, I did too." It's Friday night by the way and I'm going to have some pizza and some fun stuff, probably wings. That being said, Doug ate perfectly all the time.

Our all the time is treat your body like a temple Monday through Thursday. On Friday, treat it like a carnival. And then get right back on the wagon again. We can have a good time.

I'm going to tell one more Doug story, all right? He was going away. He was going away and it was going to be a very good time. Doug was excited to go but he was also very committed to what was going on here and he sat in front of me and says, "Boss, I'm really worried. I'm going to wreck things."

Well first of all, a year is made up of 52 weeks. He's going away for 1 weekend. He had changed his life so the exception was now something totally different. His rule had been to eat poorly, his exception was to eat cleanly. He flipped that around where his new normal was eating clean, his exception was eating poorly. That's a good equation in my world.

He went away for the weekend and he was stressed out. He comes back and he says, "I got to weight in man. I'm so freaked out." I said, "OK let's get on the scale." True story. He got on the scale, he lost 2 pounds.

He was freaking out, "Wow how does this happen?" And we'll talk about what happens in a later chapter when we talk about working out and metabolism and how we truly change the engine that runs our body. Metabolism. We have that, we'll get it out very quickly. But when that happens, that's how that happened.

He got his metabolism revved up so highly that when he was eating poorly for a weekend it really didn't do any damage. As long as he came back and got his nose to the grindstone on Monday everything was fine. That's exactly what happened.

When we need to eat well, keep it simple. 4+1 will always = 5. I purposefully made the biggest variable food. That is the single most important one. Being a gym guy, people automatically assume that working out is most important. Well it is very important and from a business perspective it's crazy important and I encourage you to come down and join our gym.

The most significant thing to changing your body, I believe, is changing your food intake. Certainly the working out part is huge as well. But you've got to put those two together. The problem we have as people is we don't want to take the time to write this down. That's the trick.

Can't Fix What You Can't See

Here's my residual story. This goes to all women. Women, I've got a secret for you. Men, they lie. All the time. Here's what I mean by that.

When I do speaking engagements, I often bring up this equation in my talk.

I say to the folks, "All right guys, this is just to the guys, who has a beer at night?"

Nobody raises their hand.

All right.

"Who has just 1?" They all raise their hand.

"Who has more than that?"

Nobody says anything, they're all lying. They have more than 1, I know it for a fact.

Let's talk about that.

If you have a light beer, we're just going to keep it simple on our calories. If you have 1 of those a week, that's 700 calories a week. You multiply that 700 times 52 weeks a year, that's a whole lot of calories that you weren't really counting for.

Truth be told when we eat chips, we're probably eating a lot more than we think. When we have pretzels, we're probably eating a whole lot more than we think. The reason I think it's significant to write it down. I'm a big fan of writing it down because I believe it becomes real. But also, you're going to realize what is wrong here.

When Doug was going through his process of figuring this out, he was a couple days into it, he walked in and threw it on my desk again and says, "I don't need you anymore, boss. I figured it out."

"What do you mean you figured it out?"

"I eat terribly."

He didn't realize that his 4 was a mess. That 4 was an 8, 9, 10, 11, 12. It was a distorted number. He didn't realize what he was eating. We don't, we just grab. We graze. We pick things up, we eat them all the time. Until we understand what we're eating, we can't fix it.

I am a firm believer, you have to take your current diet and modify it as opposed to changing everything. My suggestion? Write it down.

Figure out how many calories you're taking in. Figure out how many grams of protein. Figure out how many carbs. Figure out how many grams of fat.

Once you do that for a week or so, go back and figure out are these dense calories? Probably not.

Are they soft calories? Unfortunately, probably.

Once we then can flip those and we get a magic number, that is our magic caloric intake, we have done what so many people have tried so hard to do and that's take ownership and control of our body.

People say that all the time, "Gosh I wish I could make my body do what I want." Well truth be told you can.

I have so many clients that know, "Mike, if I take in my 2600 calories a day and I do my hour and a half of cardio a week, my body's going to be right where I want it." And they know, "Mike, during the summer I'm going to get rid of that. I'm going to do whatever I want in the summer and my body's going to change a little bit. But come fall, I'm going to go back to that."

Write down what it is that you eat. Understand what we're putting in our mouth. I talked to a gentleman the other day, he's struggling with diabetes and his blood was terrible, absolutely terrible. I was frustrated with him. He got up 2 days in a row and it was over

200. I was frustrated. I said, "Why? Why would you not fix that knowing that was a problem?" And he started talking and I was in a rant and I said, "Listen, stop. Stop." I was wrong, I probably should've let him talk, but I was frustrated. I said, "You can't control the weather. You can't control your wife. You can't control your car, your job, your work, but you know one of the very few things you can control? You can control what you put in your mouth. You have control of that number. Don't give that up."

Understand what we're putting in our mouth. And then take a look at our cardio. I'll spend a second here on cardio. Understand what you're really doing. At the gym I often see people on a say EFX cruising along. Cruise along. And this person may have done that same 3 days a week for 8 years.

Well your body's going to change to a point and then it's going to stop changing. You always do, what you've always done, you'll always get what you've always got.

So if we break this 1 down into a more specific unit, if I do cardio 3 days a week on an EFX, OK great. I challenge you. Take a look at the read out. How many strides are you doing in a 20 minutes period? How many miles are you going? Take a look at how many strides you do. And then challenge yourself. I just realized I just did 3,000 strides. OK. Next week what if you do 3,500 strides? Because now what you've done is impacted that equation yet again, which is going to force that to change as well.

Understand what you're putting in your mouth. Understand what activities you're doing and realize that that has all the influence in the world in changing what your body does. Every day.

[4]

4 For Food

4+1=5. SINCE THE BEGINNING OF TIME, that has been the case. We are going to use that math equation to illustrate how we eat. Four (4) will be the food. What we're taking in our mouth, what's going down our throat on a daily basis. One (1), is our output. What's our energy? What are we expelling every day? And five (5) illustrates the result. Even more simply put, my physical entity right now is a result of what I put in my mouth along with the activity I participate in on a daily basis. So if I change the way I eat, I'm probably going to change the way I am physically. If I change my exercise level, same thing. Now, if I change both of these units, that is going to more drastically impact who I am physically. This chapter is going to focus on the 4. The 4 is the bigger of the numbers intentionally. There is a method to my madness.

Now, I'm in the fitness business so you would think I would try to sell you on the fact that going to the gym, getting a gym membership, is the single most significant part of changing your body. I can. That would be a lie, though, because in my heart, I believe how we eat is what carries the most significance. People always come to me with, "What's the secret? What's the secret?" And quite frankly, this is what I tell them. The secret is what you do at dinner. What you do at your breakfast table. What you do at your lunch nook, or wherever it is that you eat. That's going to have the biggest impact on you changing your body. Ok, so that's probably not a good statement from a business standpoint, but it's the truth. I believe it wholeheartedly. So we're going to spend this chapter discussing the magic equation, but more specifically, talking about the number 4 – what and how we eat.

Now, before I really get started on that, I'm going to get on my soapbox and rant just a little bit. A little rant, a small rant. Here goes: So I'm in the fitness industry and people talk to me all the time about fitness goals and this and that and the other thing. On a daily basis they look at me and they go, "Mike, what's the secret? Come on. Which of those pills back there behind the bar are the ones that do it? What is the secret?" These are people who have been clients of ours at the gym for 10, even 12 years. And they still believe there's a secret. Marketers have made a lot of people a lot of money by convincing folks that there's a magic pill, or a band to put around your waist. There's a disk where you jump all around, a ball, whatever. But there is **no** magic solution.

Since the beginning of time, since humans have been on this planet, our bodies have been made up of what we eat versus, or should I say in concert with, what we do. What's our energy level? I mean, if I eat a bunch of junk and sit around and do nothing, that number is going to be pretty significantly on one side of the fence. Conversely, if I eat really well and I'm very active, chances are I'm going to be on the other side of the fence. That is what I really want to talk about, with the clear understanding that there is no magic pill or magic solution. Regardless of what a great marketer somewhere in America says, there is no magic shake that's going to change your life. Think about the word supplement; it's exactly that. It's a supplement. It should be used to supplement your diet. It shouldn't replace your diet. Our diet is what we eat on a daily basis. Again, since the beginning of time, we've been eating, running, and having a body. There were human bodies long before there were shakes, before there were pills, before there were reps, before there were all these crazy marketing concepts.

There is no magic pill. There is no magic solution. So please do your best to realize that if there is a magic solution, it's this. How you eat and how you act result in how you look. It's basic math. This is the magic pill. You want the magic pill? 4+1 will always equal 5. Always.

So let's talk about the food we put in our mouths. People often think, "well, that's not going to hurt," or "this isn't going to hurt," or "I could have a couple of those, or maybe just a few of those." If you add those little calories up over the course of a year, they can be very significant. I call them residual calories. In the first chapter, I talked in reference to gentlemen, because men lie. If you ask ladies if men lie, they're always going to say we do. So if you ask a gentleman, "hey, you have a beer at night?" He says, "Yeah, I have a beer. I have just one." Well, according to report after report, the average person who does have a beer has 2 to 2 and a half. So I'm going to use that figure here. If I have 2.5 Budweisers on a daily basis – okay, I'm going adjust that just a bit so we have a good round number to work with – if I have 2.3 Budweisers on a daily basis, that adds up to 165,000 calories a year. That's a significant number. But say we look at somebody who's been bitten by that marketing bug who subscribes to, "I'm going to get a light beer because that's a healthy option," that individual has a light beer which has 96 calories. Multiply that by 2.5, and that equals 87,000+ "residual" calories a year. Those are big numbers. It doesn't matter if it's regular beer or light beer, that is a whole bunch of calories. So if you think those "little" things are not making an impact, think again. How much of an impact is the question. This number I'm about to give you is going to cause an uproar with folks in my business, but I'm here for you, not them. So the question is, how many calories equal a pound? That number is going to change from person to person, but let's use 3,500. We can argue fewer, we can argue more, but this gives us something to work with. That being the case, if I reference the 165,000 calories for the regular beer, that's actually going to equal 47 pounds. So for that person who drinks 2.5 beers a night; if they cut that out, that's almost 50 pounds of weight loss just by getting rid of those beers which they probably didn't even think had any significance. But I've just shown you they are very significant. So the 4, which in this case is really 4 plus beer plus beer plus half a beer, is going to give me a body that's, what did I say? 47 pounds heavier? So that's going to change the numbers drastically.

Let's go back to the 4 again – and talk about me and my buddy Hudson. Hudson subscribed to the 1614 fitness lifestyle, as we like to call it, and made changes to his life. See, Hud decided that he had a goal. His goal was to drop 10 pounds, or run a 5k, or whatever the goal was. And he wanted to reach that goal by November 1st. So Hud sat down and made himself a game plan. One of the things he felt he needed to do was change his 4. He wanted to eat better. So Hudson decided what he was going to do was get up and make an egg white sandwich for breakfast every morning. He would have an egg white sandwich with a little ketchup on whole wheat toast, and that was going to be his breakfast because he knew that would be a very calorie dense, high protein breakfast. That was his game plan.

So that's what he did, and his daily intake for that meal was 232 calories. Me, I got bitten by the marketing bug. See, because I could go to a local donut shop that's known worldwide. It's got a very good marketing department. I don't know if I should name the company because I don't want to get in trouble, but let's suffice it to say that there is a very big donut shop that sells wonderful donuts and wonderful coffee which I partake of all the time. But, I decided I'm going to go there for breakfast because according to their marketing campaign, which says something like, "I'm cheating again, eating right can still taste good." I do want to eat right, because Hudson told me about his goal and I loved that goal. Hudson motivated me to also change my 4+1 because I wanted to change my body, too. I was following Hudson's lead. But, I chose not to stay home and cook. I chose to take advantage of a fairly fast food option. Because eating, what is it? Eating right still tastes good. I wanted to eat right so I ordered myself a turkey sausage sandwich with egg. I'm like, "This is good, eating right. It's turkey sausage, why not have it?"

So let's go back. Hudson was ingesting 84,000 calories a year with his breakfast. Mine, well mine was a little bit more. My turkey sandwich was 390 calories versus his 232 calories. My annual intake for breakfast was 142,000 calories. So we both knew we were making good decisions. We both knew we were manipulating the 4 in a good way, but in reality, Hudson out performed me because he decided he was going to eat his egg whites at home for 232 calories versus my going out for a donut shop breakfast sandwich with 390. So Hudson won that one hands down.

Now, let's take a look at those numbers more closely. Hudson was taking in 84,000 calories. I took in 141,000. A difference of more than 57,000 calories, or 16.5 pounds. So Hudson made better decisions. He dropped 16.5 pounds. I didn't do as well because I made a decision which was based more on marketing than what I thought would be the healthiest decision regarding breakfast. So you see how one small decision makes a big, big, big difference in our goals here. So Hudson won. He made his own sandwich; I went out and bought mine. He also probably saved more money because I spent money while he saved money. So, not only did he become more physically fit, he saved money. Which upset me because I don't want Hudson ever to win. That's never any good.

So there's a big deal in that 4 when it really didn't appear to be a big deal. Breakfast isn't that big a deal. But let's take a look at some more things that are big deals. I mentioned sausage. Again, people go, "Mike, I'm eating turkey sausage. Turkey is the white meat, it's got to be good for me, right?" Umm... Let's not say it's good for you, let's say it's better, which it is. I'm going to share with you my thoughts, which may be entirely different from yours. With that being said, let's compare pork sausage and turkey sausage. Is turkey sausage better for you? Absolutely. Is it great for you? Not so much. In fact, for my dime, I'm just going to go ahead and eat the pork sausage. I'm probably going to throw you for a loop saying that, but I would. An ounce of pork sausage has 96 calories with 2.6% saturated fat. One ounce of turkey sausage has 67 calories, with 2.3% saturated fat. Is there a difference? Absolutely. Is it big enough for me to get rid of pork sausage? Not by a long shot. So, my son and I went to a diner the other day. And he's eating, he always eats the same thing, scrambled eggs with cheese, toast, and link sausage. And you're thinking to yourself, "Wait a minute. Mike Womer, the guy who's telling me how to eat well, has a son who eats sausage?" Yep. And I eat scrapple. So anyway, my son's got his sausage. I order my eggs over easy, wheat toast, and some scrapple – because I think God wants me to eat scrapple. It's just amazing, alright? So I've got my scrapple there and my son's looking at my scrapple and asks, "Dada, what's that? I go, "That, son, is flat sausage." He says, "Flat sausage?" I go, "Yeah." He says, "Can I have some?" "Oh yeah." I give him a bite and his eyes go, boiiiiing! This is a quote, I kid you not: "Oh. That's good." Fantastic. A boy after my own heart. Okay, so I eat scrapple and sausage, yes I do. On a regular basis? No way. If I'm going to have sausage, I'm going to have pork sausage. But I'm not going to eat it very often. It's a special event when we have it. If I eat 10 meals, I expect nine of them to be healthy. That way, when it comes to the tenth, if I go out to a diner and have scrapple it's no big deal. Because this 4+1=5 thing is year long. If I have a crazy meal one day, do I just fall off the wagon? Nope, I get right back on. A piece of scrapple? Somebody may be very angry at me for saying so, but I doubt very seriously that piece of scrapple is going to kill me. Something is going to kill me one day, but I doubt it's that piece of scrapple. So do I think it's a good idea to eat turkey sausage every day? Absolutely not. Is there a difference between pork and turkey? Yes. Is it significant enough for me to eat daily? No way. So if I'm going to cheat and have fun, I'm going to cheat and have fun. I'm not going to cheat with turkey sausage. I'm going to cheat with scrapple. Because you have to get the scrapple, get the eggs – and you've got to kind of get it together – and get it on the toast. That's the way I go about it. Life is good.

So no, I don't think you have to eat 4 every day. That 4 can be a 10 now and then. Monday through Friday, I treat my body like a temple. On Saturday I've been known to have a carnival day now and then. But I do eat well 9 out of 10 days. The key is simple: understand and be accountable for what you put in your body. I probably should have said this earlier: 99% of everybody I talk to cannot give me the answer to a particular question I ask. As a matter of fact, I can only name one person who gave me the answer I was looking for. People always say to me, "Mike, tell me the secret. Tell me the secret that's going to make me be whatever number I want to be." And truth be told, I know the answer. It's rare that I know the answer to a question, but I know this one. I answer their question with, "How many calories are you taking in a day?" They give me that blank stare. "Hey, I don't know, man. Um...what day?" I don't care what day. I'm old, I can be crotchety. I don't care, dude. Until you know what that number is, we have no means of fixing it. We just don't.

When I first addressed this topic, in the previous chapter, I made the comparison of taking your car to a mechanic. You don't go in and just say, "fix it right now," without being able to tell them something about what's wrong with it. They need to know what's going on. The same thing holds true for your body. You need to know what's going on before you can make the changes you need to make in order to change your body. To figure that out, you have to document what you're eating. Back in the day, when us old people weren't so old, I would give people a book and they would write down everything they ate. Okay, so it was a pain in the duff but that's what we had to work with. Now, with smart phones, you can actually use that little scanner doo-bob and it will bump it right in and it tell you. Worst case scenario is you have type "I ate one piece of scrapple." And the phone adds it all up. It will tally it for you right now. This may, again, sound very un-Mike like. Maybe I'm not as positive as you think. We, as a society, are lazy. We're looking for that magic pill. The magic dance jump thing, lose weight, get great abs, put something around your waist. It doesn't happen. You want to be a 5, you got to do the math, okay? We already talked about Hudson eating better than I did. And he did; he out performed me because he took special care in what he was eating. I need you to do that.

Be aware of residual calories. Be cognizant of what you're putting in your mouth. We already discussed drinking light beers every day and the calories you'd take in. And we've already reviewed what eating one sandwich versus another will do.

I now want to turn the page and use a crazy word. I want to talk about glycemic index. We're still talking about what food we're putting in our mouths, but I want to talk about good foods versus very poor foods. So what is glycemic index? To really simplify it, and again, understand I'm not a nutritionist or a licensed dietitian, or anything like that. I'm just a guy who's been in business and has read more books than he probably should have on the subject. But the bottom line is, glycemic index is an indication as to how your body responds to sugars.

So let's talk about that really quick. My body has this little messenger dude who lives in my pancreas. Every time I eat sugar or anything, that little guy is down there going, "Womer's eating. He's eating bread. All right everybody, we've got to get the insulin ready. He's eating bread!" Whenever we ingest a carbohydrate, our body has to manage our sugar levels. And it does so by adjusting the insulin level. My pancreas is what facilitates that. Now, there are good carbo-

42 Yes You Can

hydrates and there are very, very bad carbohydrates. For a while, carbs were very popular. Again, I don't want to sound critical, but we get influenced too greatly by marketing.

There was a marketing craze not too long ago which pushed the idea that all carbs are bad. Carbs are terrible. Low carb diet, carb free diet, "Oh, I'm carb free!" The good Lord designed the human body to first run off of carbohydrates; secondly, run off of fats; and thirdly, run off of proteins. We will run on proteins. If we go completely carb free, our body will flick a switch. We go into ketosis, and we use proteins for our energy source. We'll do it. The body doesn't work nearly as well, but we'll do it. The fuel that we work best on is carbohydrates. It's just a fancy word for sugar. But again, there are really great carbohydrates and really bad ones. We are going to refer to the really good ones as low glycemic (good), and the bad ones as high glycemic (bad). So, let's say that I eat a piece of pumpkin pie. I'm going to eat a building full of pumpkin pie which is full of sugar and really good. When I do that, though, as soon as it goes into my gut, that little guy in my pancreas goes, "Oh boy. Oh boy. We've got sugar. Let's crank up the insulin!" As soon as I eat that the pie, my blood sugar level explodes. BOOM! That's my blood sugar spiking. Then the little man in my pancreas pushes it back down with a BOOM! of insulin. So every time I eat a simple sugar, my blood sugar goes up, but then that little guy here says we've got to push that sugar level back down. In order to do that, he cranks my body full of insulin, which shoves it right back down.

Have you ever heard the phrase, "food coma?" That explains exactly what happens. I eat the pie, my blood sugar goes up, the insulin pushes it back down, and now I'm way down here. And guess what I crave when I'm down here. My blood sugar is low so my body's like, "Oh dude. You need another piece of pie, man." So I eat another one. And my blood sugar goes right back up. And then the insulin, cranked up again, shoves it right back down. I've got this up and down going in my blood sugar all the time. A lot of people eat like this every day. But wait a minute, Mike, you said this is what happens with pie. So ... it's only pie or desserts that are high glycemic and do this? Sorry, no. That couldn't be farther from the truth. In fact, when I'm thirsty, what I like to drink is sugar water. You've never had sugar water? You've got to get on this drink. Everybody's doing it. Have you been to California recently?

Okay, first of all I've got to tell you about my cup. My son gave me this cup and there's a little spot where there's no sticker because it says "the best dad in the world," so that spot is holy. I'm not allowed to put a sticker there (I have a thing for stickers on my cups). So anyway, I'm going to drink a cup of sugar water using my dad cup. One cup. Not very much, actually. In fact, it's very little. I'm thirsty and it's really not a lot. But the part that makes it so good is the 20 grams of sugar. I love this. This is really good, you've got to try it. So how much is 20 grams of sugar? Actually, it's a lot – measure it out and see for yourself. So, why would one cup of water and 20 grams of sugar not be a good idea? If you were to go to Google and check the contents of one cup of apple juice, you'll see there are 26 grams of sugar. Think about it. One cup of water with 20 grams of sugar is absolutely insane. But if I drink apple juice, it's the same thing. Zoom! Same effect as sugar water – or pie. But it's not dessert.

Apple juice seems okay though, right?. Or maybe eat an apple. Yeah, I think an apple is the way to go. But what's the difference? But why an apple? Because the apple itself has something magical that the juice doesn't. An apple has fiber. See, apple juice is pretty much an apple with no fiber, with no substance. If I eat an apple or a better glycemic option, my body will react differently. For instance, if I drink my notorious sugar water, that is going to cause my blood sugar to skyrocket and my insulin to suppress it, and my urge will come back. I'll do it again and again, feeding that urge, and I'm up and down all over the place. Conversely, if I eat fruit or eat a very good glycemic food, the result will not be the same. One of my favorites is a sweet potato. A sweet potato is full of sugar and full of carbohydrates and full of energy, but there's a lot of fiber so it's a low glycemic food. So when I eat it, that little guy in my pancreas goes, "Uh-oh, Womer's eating a sweet potato. This is going to get nuts. Oh, wait, we'll mellow out." So he shoots some insulin but goes, "Oh, we're good. We're just going to hang here. We're okay, everything's fine." So my blood sugar and energy levels stay much more constant. I don't have the extreme ups and downs. Let's take another look at that car we took to the mechanic earlier. If I have a car, and I want it to last a long time, would I accelerate, decelerate, accelerate, slow down? Or would it just be better to cruise nice and easy? City driving versus cruising. I'll take cruising any day and the car will last longer. The same thing holds true for your body.

If I make my pancreas jump around, up and down, every day, all day for years, one day I may be sitting in the doctor's office going, "Diabetes? Really? How did that happen? Because I thought I ate well. I drink fruit juice, for crying out loud!" It's that sugar water again. It's all that sugar water. So instead of fruit juice, why not just go straight to the fruit? You know, we talked about 4+1 earlier, and I mentioned how we've been on this planet for a bazillion years, give or take a few. I sometimes think that what we did way back then was a better option than what we do now. I think sometimes the marketing and this great knowledge we've accumulated sometimes harms us. All these great sports drinks and this and that and the other thing. Aren't they very similar to sugar water? I don't want this. For the athletes that I train, and we train an awful lot of them, this is not going to provide optimal performance. In fact, my athletes are going to crash. They're going to perform at much lower levels overall than if they were nice and steady, no ups, no downs, slow and steady. Well not slow, but steady. Understand? That's big. High glycemic foods are what we don't want. And fiber keeps the glycemic levels steady. So when you look at a food and wonder what it's going to do to your blood sugar, if it will cause those ups and downs we don't want, just keep it simple. Look at the carbohydrates and then see how much fiber is in there. Is there fiber?

Here's a product that I kind of upset people with because marketing has said for years and years said that it's great for you: Yogurt. Yogurt's wonderful, yogurt's great. Yogurt does taste very good. And I think there are some great benefits to it. But here are some yogurt facts and numbers. Right now, Greek yogurt is very popular. Greek yogurt has up to 19 grams of carbs. Of those 19 grams of carbs, 12 of them are simple sugars. Do you know how many grams of fiber are in a typical tub? .5. That's right, .5. So what do you think this product is going do? It's definitely going to shoot that blood sugar up because it's got a whole lot of simple sugars. But here's what I do. I get that yogurt, I scoop it out of the container, and I put it into a bowl. Then I add a cup of raw oats and mix it up. So now all of a sudden, that simple sugar isn't so bad because I bulked it up with some fiber. So now I've manipulated that food into a much better option in terms of carbohydrates.

But again, we're not exactly go getters sometimes when it comes to this. We want it simple and easy and we love that grab and go simplicity. We love fast food. We want simple. We want the magic bullet. We want the magic tub. Again, there is no such thing. It will take effort to manipulate these numbers to give you what you're after. Speaking of that, go back and review the chapter on goals and changing your numbers. So often we think we want to be a particular 5, but once we realize how much work it takes to get there, we change our mind. We don't really want that. Really, what we're after is easy. Unfortunately, "easy" will not get you where you want to go if what you really want is to optimize your physical fitness level. If you want to avoid trips to the doctor, it will take work.

In review: residual calories count. Take a look at them, add them up. Then multiply that number by 365 and see how big that number gets. Also, be aware of the glycemic index. Simple sugars will cause highs and lows in your blood sugar. They require your pancreas to work really hard and make your body deal with increases in insulin – a lot. When we get older, that's not necessarily a good thing.

Manipulate this, manipulate that, and then you have control. And how many people really have control over their bodies? A lot of people want it and think they do, but you can have it by incorporating the steps outlined here. The equation is simple. The theory behind it is not rocket science. It's in fact very simple, and it works to a tee.

[5]

Plus One

I CAN'T POSSIBLY GET started without a little bit of a rant. Here it goes, my rant.

Four plus one equals five, I know you know what that means. We use it as an equation to help us eat better. Again, I have never been a dietitian, never been a nutritionist or any of that stuff, but I am promising you that this equation will help us eat better. It also can help us exercise more efficiently, so we can manipulate this five, which in this case if our body. My thought on this equation is this, four represents food, one represents exercise or movement, and five represents us. The way I eat combined with the way I exercise is going to give me this. Like it or not, that's just the way it works.

Here's my rant. Everybody wants to know the secret. What do I do? How do I get it? What DVD do I buy? What do I drink? There has to be a shake. There has to be a pill. There has to be some magic formula. No, not so much. That's it right there, kids. We call this at 1614 Fitness lifestyle. If you want to see some results of those lifestyles go check out our Instagram account, check us out on Facebook, or check out our website. You can see before and after pictures that were done without a magic pill, without a magic shake, without a magic DVD. It was nothing more than eating differently, exercising differently, and having a difficult body.

We've been doing it for 14 years. You can do it as well, but the problem is it takes some work. It takes some administrative effort. It takes some sweat, but man success tastes good. That's what I tell people all the time. They go, "You really are going to eat brown rice, vegetables, and lean chicken? Really? Does that taste good?" I go, "I think it taste okay, but I think the success I feel when I achieve my goal tastes better than any cake, or any cookie, or anything like that." That may sound silly, but when I have a goal I have goal, and I encourage you to check out the other episodes on goal because I go into huge, big time rant about just how important our goals are. I'll touch on it a little bit.

If your goal is to be a five, I mean really to be a five, and you've gone through and validated just how important that five is, you can achieve that five if that's what you want. I encourage you to spend some quiet time, figure out what your goals are, figure out how important they are, then you can move forward. That being said, enough of my rambling.

Four plus one equals five, four is food. It's bigger. One is exercise, let's talk about that. Exercise. I'm a firm believer in quantifying as much as I can because I feel as though if I get a benchmark on something and I understand it, I then have the wherewithal to make an educated decision on how to manipulate it to give me the result I want. I say it all the time. I can't fix a car's engine without evaluating the problem.

I need to know not only what I'm eating from a caloric perspective, a protein perspective, a carbohydrate perspective, a fat perspective, a lot, but I need to know what I'm doing from an exercise perspective. I need to get my arms around that. I'm going to share some stories on how we can do that, and some experiences I've had as a trainer on how I've witnessed that.

In this era, there's a couple ways we can track our intensity or our workload or volume. We're going to talk about those two words in a little bit. There're two ways of doing it. Very clearly, we can an electronic device to do it, or we can do it manually.

Let's talk about the electronic device. I should devices. There're a lot of mechanisms, device, little computers that we can wear as a watch that'll track how many calories we burn, how many steps we take. There's a lot of those very, very cool devices. There's also the old school way of writing it down. I'm going to talk a lot about that here in a second. Let's go back to electronic.

I see a lot of people in the gym, and when the come into the gym they put on their gear, they do this, and they put on their timepiece that's really the calorie counter, which is great. I think that needs to be looked at with a bigger view, a bigger picture. If I come into the gym and I have my electronic device on and I know I burn 500 calories, big round number, keep it simple, 500 calories.

Do I know if that's good? Do I know if that's bad? I don't know. I would much rather have a person wear that electronic device on a regular basis so they can see how many calories they burn as a whole or every day. What's their average? Let's wear that device for a month. Let's figure out what our average caloric burn is. Let's take a look at how many strides we're taking.

Then, if that's our baseline, if our baseline is 3,500 calories and we want to manipulate it, now we know we can start with a goal. Maybe our goal is 3,800 calories, 4,200 calories. I'm just pulling numbers out of my head. We know what we can do to manipulate that. Again, I think if we're going to use the electronic device, figure what we're doing on a daily basis, just not for those two hours we're working out. I think that can skew the number a little bit.

I'm a big fan of going old school. It allows me to look at it, but again, we have apps now. I have a lot of clients who use MyFitnessPal, and I can log on and see what they're doing. I guess I'm converting slowly to the electronic. It's just a hard thing for me to do. Manually, I use a lot with my clients still.

What we do is we just track what you do on a daily basis, so I can look at it. I may very often, I don't may, I do on a very regular basis give homework to my clients. Chuck hates me right now because I'm asking him to give him 25,000 strides a week. That doesn't make any sense now but it will in a second, so hold on.

I like to track manually. More times than not, I'm going to track our cardio, not so much our resistance training. That's a little bit different. I want to know what our cardio output is. That being said, remember I like baselines, I'm going to call them Steve. Steve has been a wonderful client and wonderful friend for a long time.

He walked into the gym four years ago and looked me very clear in the eye and says, "My name is Steve, and I'm going to change my life. I'm going to get fit. I'm going to do it starting now." I hear that all the time. Not so much, but to Steve's credit, not only has he lost 50-ish pounds. He went from somebody who never consider running, he's an avid runner now. He does 5Ks on a regular basis. You can see him on Instagram. He's going to be the gentleman holding the pants out that used to be way too big. That's Steve.

Here's Steve's story. Steve came into the gym, and said, "I'm going to lose weight right now and you're going to help me." We set up an appointment. We got together. We did a consult. We did the evaluation, his fat body, and all that good stuff.

We got an EFX machine. That's a just simple elliptical machine made by Precor. We use them all the time. It's a great piece. A lot of people have them in their homes.

He got on this device and I said it very simply. I didn't do any manipulation. I said, "Get on, Steve. Let's see what we have." I think he lasted two and a half minutes. He was not happy. He's like, "I didn't even last five minutes." I quickly grab my pen, wrote myself a love note. Steve lasted two and a half minutes, slobbering, sweating, snotting. He was a mess, but that was our benchmark.

That's where we started.

From that moment, I started to document manually what Steve did. To this day, every single day Steve does cardio, every day he texts me on my phone, "Mike, ran a quarter mile, man this." Every single thing he does he sends me to this day. It gives him accountability. He mails me his cardio output, not only for my sake but for his sake. He needs to know. Again, he succeeded. If it ain't broke, don't break it. Steve keeps sending me those pieces of information, man, because you're doing great. We keep track of that.

Here's what I may do. I say, "Steve, we lasted two and a half minutes. Great job. We have to start somewhere. Our next goal is going to be three minutes." Maybe our next goal is going to be five minutes. Before you know it, we're cranking things up. We're 10, we're 15, before you know it, we're 20 minutes into this thing. Before long, Steve was able to get on the EFX machine and cruise for 20 minutes. Put that on hold. Everything on hold for five seconds because here's ... I guarantee you somebody watching this right now is going, "This dude's crazy, man, if he thinks I'm going to get on one of those crazy spinning devices and spin my butt for 20 minutes. Way too bored for that."

You're right, dude. Nobody on this planet is shorter attention span than I. if I was kid now I would have ADHD, I'd have ADD, I'd have KFC, I'd have every ESPN. I'd have them all. If you know me a little bit, you know I'm a spaz, so dude, I know. You have to figure out what you need to do to make cardio work. I blindly watch the video noise, the TV screen, but I'm always listening to music, and I sing along, I do whatever it takes. People next to me go, "That cat's crazy." I am, but if it ain't broke, don't fix it. That's what works for me.

I make music lists and I listen to them. Sometimes they're hard and fast, sometimes they're slow and mellow. Everything's different.

I do what I have to do to get me through that cardio. Okay, that little report's done. Let's go back to Steve.

Now he's back. He has himself back to 20 minutes of cardio. He's losing weight. He's doing great. He is just rocking out. Steve thinks we're just going to continue to tack on this cardio duration. He's like, "Dude, before long I'm going to be at 75 minutes." Wait a minute, as a trainer can I really ask my client to just keep doing more and more and more and more cardio? From an athletic nutrition, many reasons, that's not a great idea. Just from a life perspective, eventually I have to stop doing more because I have a life to lead. I can't do an hour of cardio every day. I can't do 75, 80 minutes of cardio a day. I have to make some changes.

Here is where I change up and diversify a little bit. We're going to start with volume training, meaning I'm going to add more volume. Then, we may have to change gears and go into intensity based, and we may very well go back to volume. I'm a firm believer, our body will change and make adjustments based on its workload.

When Steve went from doing two and a half minutes to doing 10, 15, we upped the volume. His body changed. He burned additional calories. He lost what. He toned up. If I don't make change to his workout routine his body will stop changing. If we now do four plus two equals six, and I don't change that it's now become two, if I don't change that some more he'll always be a six. Steve pays me for this to improve all the time, so I need to make constant change to this. Therefore, I will toggle back and forth to keep his workouts changing. If you always do what you've always done you'll always get what you've always got. Grammatically, it's a disaster, but from an exercise perspective, it's accurate. Think about that again.

If you always do what you've always done, you'll always get what you've always got. It's simple. I need to change this and/or that, or preferably both, I make big changes to that five. Here's what we do with this volume change with Steve. I was messing around with him and he didn't even know it.

Steve would come in. I'd say, "Hi, buddy. Let's just do your five minutes. Do your five minutes of cardio like you always do." He and I are going to do chest and back or whatever we're going to do that day. He gets off of it. We workout. I say, "Steve, listen, do me a favor. I want you to jump back on the treadmill, but I have a goal." He has no idea what's going on at this point. He thinks I'm incorporating some split, some cross training, some crazy thing. Really, I'm screwing with him by gathering data.

Here's what I'm doing. When he did his first five minutes on that device the Precor EFX will count strides. It'll tell me how many strides he's averaging per minute. It'll also tell me how many total strides he does in a 10-minute, five-minute, seven-minute duration. What I've done, Steve's doing his five, I'm watching. Five minutes, total strides, and then I figure out his average stride.

I say, "Okay, Steve, I know you're carrying 200 strides a minute. That's the pace you were able to keep. I'm going to add five, 10 strides a minute, times it by 10, and say, "Here's a little sticky. I'm going to put the sticky. Steve, I want you to do 2,100 strides as quickly as you can." Listen, if somebody has a goal and they had to stick-to-it'edness to achieve that goal the way Steve does, if you put a little sticky pad and put if on the EFX, that little board there, and say, "I want you to hit that number as quickly as you can," he's like, "I have to get to 2,100. I have to get to 2,100. I have to get to 2,100. I got it, nine minutes and 13 seconds."

What I've done, I've screwed with Steve's intensity. Didn't even know it. I can't increase volume all day long because I'm going to run out of daylight. Eventually, you just have too much. Too much of a good thing is too much. I have to mess with is intensity.

See, ultimately it goes back to this number again. I'm trying to manipulate this number. See, now we were four plus two equals six, but now I've increased his intensity over a long period of time, now we're four plus three equals seven. All of a sudden, Steve's like, "This guy's a genius." Not really. All I'm doing is incorporating what we like to call at 1614 Fitness lifestyle. It's not rocket science. We're just manipulating what he's putting in his mouth and what he's doing from an exercise perspective. He's changing his body. Steve will be the first to tell he didn't change that a whole lot. He eats better than he did, but he has a good time.

I've gotten texts from him two, three, four in the morning as if it's nothing. Boy, I'm telling you what, you want to see a success story, Steve's your guy. Day in, day out. He lives, breathes, and eats the 1614 Fitness lifestyle.

We can measure volume a lot of different ways. We can measure volume, number of strides, if you're using a device. We can measure volume on how long you went, how far you traveled. If you're going to do volume and you're going to do it outside, how far you went on a track. When the weather's nice go outside. Two miles is two miles.

Then again, once you reach a certain point, typically I use the 20-minute barrier is my mark. When I have a client who have 20 minutes fairly comfortably, instead of going to 25 minutes, or 30, or 35, I tend to start working on intensity. They're using an EFX product where I know what their average strides are. I get out the calculator. I say, "Right now you're averaging 185 strides."

I don't tell them this because I'm trying get them to do more than they want. I go and I get on a calculator. You're average 187 strides. You're great. I want to increase their intensity, so let's go 195. Where'd I get that number? I just made it up. You just pull a number, see if you can get it. Make it achievable, but see if you can get it.

Now I'm going to change your average from 187 strides per minute, or whatever I said a second ago, to 195. Then, I'm going to times that by 10 or 15 or whatever that magic number is and I'll write it down on a sticky. "All right, kiddo, there it is, 1,700 strides." Again, I just pulled that number out. See if you can beat in under 10 minutes or whatever that figure is. You're going to increase the intensity, and you're going to be able to crank it out.

Then, I may say, "Great. You can average 210 strides. That's awesome." You've showed me that you can do that for 12 minutes. Now toggle back to volume, now let's see if you can carry that for 15 minutes. I'm going to ask you to increase your intensity, but now I'm going to ask you to carry it over a longer period of time. Now at the end of the day we have increased their volume and their intensity which is going to have a greater impact on this.

This is all, I think, logical, and I think simple. The problem is do you have the ability to stick with it? Again, all of these before and after pictures that we have on our various sites they are people that did, that flat out had that ability. Steve is a wonderful example, because I'm telling to this day ... Steve was in Florida. On two occasions while he was in Florida I got texted. He was in the hotel workout room and he sent it to me. He sent me a little piece of it, something, I saw this on a piece of equipment I thought you'd want to know. Dude, that is absolutely stellar.

He's not bananas. He spent 20 minutes running, so it's not like he hurt his vacation. Again, I'm not telling you to always workout on your vacation, I'm not. I'm just giving you an example of a person who thoroughly has a great case of stick-to-it'edness. I don't think that's a word, but we're going to use it right now because that's what's enabled him to lose that what, and to more importantly to keep that weight off. He truly has changed his lifestyle.

He did not incorporate a diet. He did not engage in a fast. He did not engage in any of these kick-start programs. He didn't decide to drinking shakes or getting a disk where you jump up and down and roll tires over on it. He just changed his lifestyle, and he's done a great job of it. He's not a five by any stretch of the imagination because he has recognized what his number is, he tracked it manually, we manipulated his volume, then his intensity, then we married the two together, and it worked. It continues to work for him and continues to work for many other folks.

I encourage you to take a step back and see what do you do. Do I sit at home and do very little? That's not terrible. That makes it easy quite frankly. Because if I have a client who eats poorly and doesn't anything, we're going to achieve some good success by doing very little. If I have somebody who's sitting at home and not exercising a lick, if I can get them to come to the gym or go outside and walk 20 minutes three times a week, you carry over the course of a month, carry that over the course of a year, that's whole lot different. That's not a one anymore. That's a significant bump. I hope that change that they see wets their appetite enough like it did with Steve, like it did with countless other people where they go, "This is great."

I think people sometimes look at fitness people and exercise people with a little bit of ... there's just not just favorable all the time. I think sometimes people look at fitness people as people who might think they're better than others. Not so much here. Or somebody who thinks that they can do more things, and I'm going to live forever because I had a person say that to me once. They said, "Mike, what do you think? You're going live forever? Why do you do all this fitness stuff?"

No, I may not live a day longer, but pretty sure I'm going to have more fun in the time I have because I'm 47 years old. I'm creeping on 50. I [inaudible 00:20:26] that, but my goal other than things that are really important, my goal is to have a lot of fun, to be able to do things with my son, to be able to run up and down stairs without being totally winded. The only way I do that is to keep moving.

Four plus one always equals five. Always will, always has, and will always. Four is my food, one is my exercise, five is me. If I want to manipulate that five, manipulate the exercise, manipulate the food, and I will change that I absolutely guarantee it.

Programmed to Succeed

TODAY I WANT TO TALK about a couple of things. I want to very much want to drive home the fact that you gotta have a goal. We're going to talk about physical placement and that's a weird combination or words, but we're going to make it make sense in just a few moments. We're going to talk about schedule and that sounds overly simple, but we're going to make it relevant. Finally, do you like it? It's not what you think, so stay tuned.

What is exercise? Well, In my world, exercise is very simply put. It's movement. If you're sitting sanitary, you're not exercising, you're not moving. So, what is it? It's moving around and it doesn't have to be in a gym. It doesn't have to be on monkey bars or any of that kind of stuff. It can be as simple as playing basketball, walking dog, playing with your child, body boarding at the beach, playing tennis, playing basketball at a church group. It could be a lot of different things. In my mind, exercise is movement.

What's going on in our world, however, is that people realize that you can make an awful lot of money through exercise. I've proved to my account day in and day out that I'm not one of those guys, but a lot of people are very successful in making money. How do they do it? They market their movement better than other companies market their movement.

So what I'm talking about is, you can go to Cross Fit, you can get an online thing, you can Insanity, you can get, I think there's a Beach Body thing out there. You can do a lot of different programs, all of which very much have a place in the fitness world. But, are they for everybody at this point, this time? Probably not and I want to talk about that. I'm gonna bring these items, kind of see if they fit. There I think is the crux of the problem. These workout programs don't fit for everybody in their current placement. So, are they good? Absolutely, they're good. In fact, they're great for some people, but not everyone. So, let's start there. What do you need to insure that your program works? First thing you gotta do, is you have to have a goal. Now, that being said, I encourage you to go back to our second in our series of Exercise for Beginners. We have an episode entirely dedicated to goal setting. How to bring a goal to life, how to convert it from being a win to a goal, what do you do to make it work and how do you exceed those goals.

We have an entire episode and I encourage you to check that one out. It's actually my favorite because I believe in life, whether it's fitness, whether it's relationships, whether it's a job, setting a clear goal is going to help you get there. I don't think you have a shot at doing it really, without a clear goal. So, make sure you have a goal in your fitness world. So, I say that if you don't have a goal, how can you possibly establish a work out routine that's going to get you there? You need to know where you're going. You need to say, listen, is my goal to run a 5K? Is my goal to lose X amount in inches? Is my goal to be better conditioned so I can play with my child? Is my goal to lower my cholesterol? Once you establish that goal, now you're in a position to make an educated decision on which fitness program works for you. So many times I hear people say, "I gotta get in shape. Such a generic phrase. I gotta get in better shape" and they go, "Okay, I'm going to choose that workout routine." That workout routine may not be the best option, which leads us to 2, 3, and 4. You can't go to 2, 3 and 4 without 1. You gotta get yourself a goal and it's gotta be a concise goal and 1 more plug. Go back to our episode, Setting Goals. I think it will help. This plays a big, big, big role in 2, 3, and 4, all right? So we've got the goals squared away. You know exactly what it is, when it's going to be achieved.

Now, physical placement. That's a weird phrase, physical placement. In fact, we were talking about it earlier, do we want to change that? Do we want to change that to physical condition and we chose not to because you can have different kinds of condition.

You can have a condition meaning, I'm in great physical condition. I can run 10 miles. I can't do 5 push ups, but I can do 10 miles. Conversely, you can be in condition where you can do a whole bunch of physical activities, like push ups, but couldn't run a 5K. SO, condition is too vague. I want physical placement. Here's what I mean by that: If I have a newbie, who comes into our gym, 1614 Fitness, and is de-conditioned; it's a mom or grandmom or a dad or an uncle who isn't involved in any physical activity right now, other than just their normal life. Maybe they walk at the mall once a week or something of that nature and they say, "I'm going to do box jumps. I'm going to get in a cage and do a push press. I want to go to hang cleans or I want to go do dumbbells, or I'm going to go get on a BOSU." This is not a good idea. They're physical placement is not conducive to that dynamic environment.

All right, dynamic environment, what do I mean? Well let's start off, if those folks would come into the gym and I would give them a tour and they say, "I want to do it. Let's get squared away." I would give them a very detailed, organized workout routine that would be very much in the beginning.

All I want you to do is get familiar with machines, A, B, C, D, and F. Perfect.

In a perfect world, these folks will continue to work out and will progress, enabling me as a trainer to incorporate progressions. Pretty logical, but a lot of people ignore that.

So, what's a normal progression?

Well, we can increase a number of...or their resistance, we can increase the number of sets. So, now they're getting stronger. But when you're doing those machines, most of them are unilateral. I'm in 1 of these machines and I don't need to stabilize anything. The machine is doing an awful lot of that work.

So, as an athlete, and I use that word on purpose, because if you're in a gym or outside and you're working out and you're training, you're an athlete. Maybe not a world class athlete, maybe you're not an Olympic athlete, but you're an athlete and we're going to treat you like one.

So, now, this machine no longer challenges me, so next progression could be, what if we go on a weight loaded isolateral machine, where now I've got to keep up both hands.

Maybe to the next progression would be to do free weights. Maybe the next progression would be dumbbells. Maybe the next progression would be going into the studio and doing BOSU exercises, balance, incorporating bands and all that good stuff. That's a conversation for another day, but I want you to understand that their place, physically needs to play a huge role in where they work out, how they work out and which exercise program they chose. That placement is absolutely crucial. Again, do I want a newbie to go out and do box jumps, hang cleans, push presses? Absolutely not. I need them to get stronger in the core. If I had a dollar of every coach that told me when I was young, "Son, you gotta work on your core, son, you gotta work on your core, son, you gotta work on your core", I would be buying all of us right now. That being said, we don't do a good job of that as a whole. Those machines, that I was making fun of myself, there is machines typically are not going to help you get stronger in that area. As we progress, and do more challenging motions, forcing us to get stronger, now all of a sudden, as that progression continues, now we can start doing things like box jumps, hang cleans and all that sort of thing.

1 of the first things I do, now I'm going to come across a salesperson in this. In a perfect world, all folks who are interested would go to a gym, 1614, gotta love that plug and go grab themselves a trainer and go get an evaluation so they can figure out where they are. So then they can get a professional person to help guide them in that selection.

Here's something I do with athletes all the time. Now, we're going to, as we get into this series or addition of series, I'm going to have examples of exercises. But, I'm going to give you a tidbit. I will do an assessment on an athlete. I'm going to look at their posture; I'm going to see if they can do an athletic position. I'm going to see if they can do a static squat; I'm going to see they can do a dynamic squat and if they can do those, I'm going to send them over here. If they can't do those correctly, I'm going to send them over here and chances are, they're going to be somewhere in the middle and which means I'm going to put them somewhere here. So, again, if you were in a position where you can go to a gym, have a consultation...most gyms, 1614 does it free all the time, get yourself a trainer, and do a free consultation, figure out where you are physically, and then align yourself with the most appropriate workout program. That to me, is crucial. But again, that trainer needs to know your goal, so they can combine those 2 items to make a selection.

Now, we've got 2 of those elements done. Now we've got to move on to this 1, which seems very simple. You're going to say, "Well Mike, if it fits in my schedule, it's good. If it doesn't, it doesn't." Yeah, no kidding. You're absolutely right, but here's what I see people doing all the time. They bite off a little bit more than they can chew. So, they say, "All right, I got a goal. I want to run a 5K. I want to do it in 3months. This guy Mike Womer did this episode and I decided I'm going to do that." Then, I went to 1614 Fitness, Allen, otherwise known as NASCAR, gave me a free evaluation and said this is my suggestion. So, I followed Allen's suggestion. I'm going to work out. In fact, I'm going to work out with my partner. We're going to work out because, see, 1614 Fitness opens at 5:30 every day. We're going to get together every other morning at 5:30 and work out. Fantastic, I hear people say that all the time and it works for 2 or 3 weeks and then they realize, dude, I'm not much of a morning person, tired. That being said, that morning routine doesn't work really well, or somebody says, you know what I'm going to do? I'm going to go to work, I'm going to go home, have dinner with my family, I'm going to put my child to bed, then I'm going to come in at 8:30, 9:00. That's what I'm going do. Well, they do that and by 9:00, they go, give me time out. I need a moment. I'm tired. I'm going to go to bed. It doesn't work. It doesn't fit in their routine. Where another fellow may say, I got an hour and 15 minutes for lunch. If I speed down there, get all the lights, I can get a shower, come back and I'm good. Well, again, something goes wrong. It doesn't fit. We have to find a workout that fits your schedule. Sure, there's going to be times when it doesn't work perfectly, but it has to fit somewhat comfortably or you're not going to stick to it. What I'm getting at with this 1 is if it doesn't stick, it's not going to work. You can have a world class fitness program designed, you can have a great goal, you can have a fitness professional design it and lead you on the way, but if your schedule doesn't fit that, it's not going to work. Maybe your better option is to walk before work, walk after work. Maybe you can walk during work. Maybe you can have a church league to play basketball. I don't know, but I think you've got to find these things, funnel them into a more specific opportunity and go with it. You got to make sure you've got a goal. You got to make sure you know where you are physically, and if it doesn't fit in your schedule, it's just not going to work and people, I see people take a monster bite and say "I'm going to be there at 5:30." Well, I'm there at 5:30 a lot. I get up everyday at 4:30. It's not a big deal to me. I get up normally without an alarm clock thing. I turn it off. So, that's no big deal but people say, I'm going to do that. That being said, we've been open for almost 14 years. I've seen some of the same folks day in and day out and God bless them. But if it doesn't work for you, don't commit to it because it won't work.

Now, this is the one everyone giggles at. Do you like it? Do you like it? I don't mean, do you like this workout routine like you like happy hour. I don't mean do you like this work out routine like you like a puppy or a kitten, because you're not going to. There's a small group of folks that love working out. They love to tingle and spark of endorphins. I love it, but not everybody does. Some folks, they come to me and they say, "Mike, listen, I have no desire to work out." We'll call this guy, Kurt. Kurt's at the gym right now. It's not really his name, and everybody knows it, but he came to us and he got a hold of 1 of our trainers. His name is Mike Dalton. They call him Chop. I don't know why we call him Chop, but we do. Kurt, I got to remember his alias. Kurt has no desire to work out. He's de-conditioned, but his doctor is going bananas. You need to work out. Your blood levels are here. Your sugar are here. You're not good. So, he will flat out tell you, "Mike, I don't like working out." But, I talked to him 2 days ago and his blood levels are astronomically better. He says, "Mike, I'm probably never going to like working out, but I'm probably never going to stop, either." So, I think that's a blessing. See, you don't have to like it, like it, but what I want you to do is I want you to quantify it, all right? I want you to quantify how much you dislike it. That being said, I need your goal. Let me rephrase that. You need your goal to have a greater value than the amount you dislike working out. What I mean is, working out is down here, but my goal is here. Does this weigh enough to bring it here? It does with Kurt and I pray it always does.

Here's a funny story. A gentleman came into the gym, it could be 10 years ago, who knows, and he said talk to me about memberships and I'm kind of in a tenuous position because I come across at times as a salesperson, but he walked in the door and asked...he said,

"Hey, listen, I need a gym membership."

So, I said, "Well, you can do this, you can do that, or if you really want to do this, there's a 3 month membership." I want to do that. So, let me get this straight, sir. You want to do that, 3 months. Yes. You want to get in shape for 3 months? Yes. So, you don't want to be in shape the 4th month and he looked at me and he's like, what do you mean?

I go, "Isn't this a life style? Doesn't it make more sense to commit that this is what you're going to do 2 to 3 times a week? So you want to be in shape January, February, March, but not so much April, May, June. I don't recall what he did, but I remember he looked at me as if I was crazy.

He says, "I don't understand." I do. I believe that physical activity needs to reoccur all the time. The good lord designed our body to run and we sit down, we start to break down and that's problematic.

So, we've got to make...we've got to find 1 that we like enough to continue, all right? Steps to success here, I think are pretty simple. We need to find a work out routine that will satisfy our goal, it will clearly satisfy our goal. There's a ton of good ones out there. I talked about those ones earlier. They're fine. They're fantastic for a lot of people. They make a lot of people happy. They make a lot of people fit and they make a lot of people money.

God bless ya. But, your goal needs to make sense with the exercise program you select, your physical placement. This 1 might be the most important because this is the 1 that can get you hurt. A prerequisite. You've got to have a whole bunch of prerequisites before you can go to any major university and take Chem 2. All right.

The same should be true about working out. If you can't stabilize your body to do X, Y, and Z, you better not go progressive, do other things, until you're ready. That's what a meeting with a fitness professional, I think, makes the best sense. Again, I'm going to come across as a salesperson, but it's logic, isn't it? If you can't do a very simple exercise, do you jump on a box, do squats? I don't think so. I think it's a poor decision and just begging to get hurt.

Scheduling, if it doesn't fit in your schedule, it's not going to last. It goes back to that 3 month deal, if it's not going to last, why do it? I've had a lot of people say, "Hey, Mike, listen. I've got my membership. I'm going to continue to come, but I may take a break in the summer because I want to get outside and do things, because it's just fun." God bless you, man, go do it. You got to find something that you're going to stick with.

Exercise programs fail because here. They also succeed because here. Make sure you set a goal. Find out where you are physically, make it fit in your schedule, and find 1 that you enjoy, at least a little bit. Maybe not as much as puppies, but make sure you enjoy it.

ABOUT THE AUTHOR

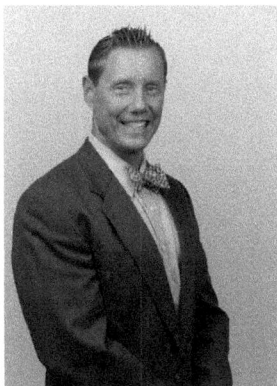

Mike Womer, as seen on CNN, ABC, CBS, FOX, NBC and FOX News, is a nationally recognized fitness expert, performance coach, personal trainer, fitness club owner and motivational speaker who inspires through his high energy delivery and passion for life. He created 1614 Fitness in Bear, Delaware in 2001 and developed 1614 Speed and Agility in 2006. Mike has trained three Delaware High School State Championship Teams, Wilmington University athletic teams, several of the region's top travel squads, a professional triathlete and has consulted with multiple athletes as they prepare for pro day and workouts with prospective professional teams.

Mike has travelled across the country to facilitate speaking engagements to multiple top Fortune 500 Companies. He continues to present his acclaimed "1+4=5" eating series throughout the Delaware Valley and speaks to local businesses regarding nutrition, health and goal setting.
Mike has been married to Sandy for 7 years and together they raise their 6 year old son, Jacob.

To learn more about Mike and 1614 Fitness, go to 1614fitness.com or follow them on Facebook and Instagram

www.ingramcontent.com/pod-product-compliance
Lightning Source LLC
Chambersburg PA
CBHW070840300326
41935CB00038B/1306